HEALTHY HABITS SYSTEM WORKBOOK

by

Corey S. Jackson, MS
Nutrition, CPTL3,
Weight Management
Specialist

Information presented in the workbook is not intended as a substitute for the medical advice of physicians. The reader should regularly consult their doctor in matters relating to his/her health and particularly with respect to any symptoms that may require diagnosis or medical attention. Please confer with your physician before beginning any nutrition, supplement, or exercise program to ensure that you are healthy enough to do so. Any sport involving speed, equipment, balance and environmental factors poses some inherent risk. The author advises readers to take full responsibility for their safety and know their limits. Before practicing the skills described in this book, be sure that your equipment is well maintained, and do not take risks beyond your level of experience, aptitude, training, and comfort level.

HEALTHY HABITS SYSTEM WORKBOOK by Corey S. Jackson published by Pretty Good Planners, 5401 S. FM 1626 Suite 170-192, Kyle, TX 78640

www.PrettyGoodPlanners.com

First printing: 2017

TABLE OF CONTENTS

HEALTHY HABITS SYSTEM WORKBOOK 1

PREFACE 7

INTRODUCTION 11

PART 1: DO 20

CHAPTER 1: EDUCATE 24

CHAPTER 2: EVALUATE 26

CHAPTER 3: CREATE 28

PART 2: EDUCATE 37

CHAPTER 1: EAT 39

CHAPTER 2: DRINK 48

CHAPTER 3: MOVE 52

CHAPTER 4: SLEEP 61

PART 3: EVALUATE 66

CHAPTER 1: EAT and DRINK 70

CHAPTER 2: MOVE 72

CHAPTER 3: SLEEP 75

PART 4: CREATE 78

CHAPTER 1: EAT 80

CHAPTER 2: DRINK 90

CHAPTER 3: MOVE 94

CHAPTER 4: SLEEP 96

CHAPTER 5: TROUBLESHOOTING YOUR PLAN 100

DO YOUR PLAN 105

EPILOGUE: 107

WHAT NEXT? 107

RE-EVALUATE 109

RECALIBRATE. 113

PREFACE

What you can expect the next five weeks

Habits Lead, Results Follow
 - Corey Jackson

THIS WORKBOOK is part of a 5-week program that teaches you how to develop healthy habits that can lead to lasting results for your fitness and your life.

Throughout this book, there are references to workbook material. You'll be able to see in this book how some of the worksheets are laid out, but you might want to print out a copy of the full set of pages so you have a head start.   To do that, go to. https://www.clearpathfitness.com/healthy-habits-system-free-download. That will give you a free set of digital workbook pages to use with this book.

You may notice that the downloads are at the website for Clear Path Fitness. Since publishing this book, I have started an online training business that is changing lives and giving people the tools that they need to succeed with their fitness and nutrition. I invite you to explore and find out more while you're there.

Your Healthy Habits Schedule

Week 0:

- Day 0.1: Educate
    - Eat
    - Drink
    - Move
    - Sleep
- Days 0.2-0.3: Evaluate your habits now
- Day 0.4: Create your goal and plan for the next four weeks
    - Eat – menu and grocery list
    - Drink – hydration strategy
    - Move – workout schedule
    - Sleep – Sleep Booster™ routine
- Days 0.5-0.7 – Coordinate
    - Track before photos, measurements
    - Grocery shop, pre-cooking
    - Buy large water bottle
    - Make workout arrangements
    - Build optimal sleep environment

Week 1 (Days 1-7): Track and Execute

Week 2 (Days 8-14): Track and Execute

Week 3 (Days 15-21): Track and Execute

Week 4 (Days 22-28): Track and Execute

- Day 28: Reevaluate
    - After photos, measurements
    - Goal reset

The Healthy Habits System™ at a glance:

DO
- Each week has 168 hours
- Daily activities should support life goals
- Enjoy the journey, but know where you're going

EAT
- Whole, unprocessed foods
- Proper portions
- Planned and prepped meals and snacks

DRINK
- Water first
- (Bodyweight/2) ounces of water each day
- Add 8 ounces for every coffee/tea/alcohol

MOVE
- Strength, cardio, flexibility that grow with you
- According to YOUR fitness level
- Do something you LOVE every day

SLEEP
- Restorative sleep is integral to optimal fitness
- Good restorative sleep starts in the morning
- Sleep Booster rituals result in restorative sleep

INTRODUCTION

You can always do more than you think you can. You are more capable than you have ever dreamed!
- Corey Jackson

HAVE YOU EVER tried to put a puzzle together without the benefit of a guiding image? Or maybe you know what it should look like, but there are the wrong number of pieces in the box? Imagine getting the puzzle put together, yet finding several pieces left over. What do you do with them?

For many, these analogies describe adding the daily tasks of getting fit and losing weight to their already full lives. They know they need to lose weight, but they don't know what they need to do to lose it, nor do they know how to organize their lives so that they can focus on it while staying effective in every other area. They don't have a reference image of what their day/week/month should look like on the way to achieving their fitness goals.

Yet others may know what they need to do to get fit but find that their daily lives present too many pieces. Putting their puzzle together is like trying to fit rocks of varying sizes into a cylinder; if it's done in the wrong order, there will be rocks left over after the cylinder is full. And while their health is important to them, the other pieces are not optional parts of their schedule, so they find that, more often than not, the daily work of weight loss gets left out of the schedule.

Even others have put in the work and have lost the weight, but without an appealing daily framework for continuing the work, they have let the busy-ness of their lives take over and have lost their results. Let me ask you: Do you see yourself in one of those scenarios?

If so, you are not alone. In fact, according to a study published in The Lancet in 2016[1], almost one-third of the world's population was considered overweight or obese. I'm sure you've heard this statistic characterized as an 'obesity epidemic'. And while society tends to characterize the overweight as lazy, you know you're not lazy – how can you be with all you do? Likewise, it's unreasonable, and unrealistic, to label nearly 30% of the entire world as lazy. You're a high-achieving person with big goals, big dreams, and big responsibility. You are successful, capable, and driven at whatever you do. Whether you're in business, or law, or public service; whether you're a creative, a student, or in charge of growing humans – or any combination of (any or all) of those things – you have too much going for you to even think you're lazy. You simply have too many pieces of the puzzle left over after you've completed your picture.

Or so it seems. But the truth is, everyone has the same number of pieces. For every person on the planet, every week contains 168 hours. While the circumstances of every person's life are unique, we all have the same amount of time to do something with our circumstances. If you're struggling to make self-care a high enough priority that it doesn't get pushed out of your schedule, it's not because you have less time than anyone else, nor is it because you have been given a box with too many pieces. You simply need a framework that informs how you put the pieces together.

Why habits are important

Let's return to the third scenario, in which you have lost weight and gained it back. While many of us have successfully lost weight, research[2] shows that less than 20% of us have maintained our weight loss successes.

That means that more than 80% of those that have intentionally spent time, money, and effort on losing weight and transforming their shape and health have lost those changes. We're not just imagining it; research has borne out the fact that most people that lose weight gain it back, sometimes with extra pounds for good measure. Those numbers intrigue me as a wellness professional. And while many researchers look at the metabolic underpinnings of weight loss reversal to explain the failure of the 80%, I began looking closer at what made the 20% successful. I wanted to know what they knew, so I could help as many as possible join their ranks.

All the data gathered suggest that the difference between the 20% and the 80% can be reduced to one thing: *Habit.*[2]

Your habits can make you successful, or they can make you fail. Habits can set you free or they can ensnare you. Habits are the main thing that we all have in common; whether those habits bring us to victory or defeat depends on their nature. This is true in every facet of your life, not just what you do or don't eat.

Why a physical planner?

So many things are done digitally now, why would you want a physical planner, with pages to write on and turn, when there's an app for that? Lots of research has been done on the neuroscience of learning that points to the necessary role of writing in the process.

The actual physical activity of putting pen to paper literally makes a neurological difference by mapping new neuronal connections between regions responsible for intention, learning, and motor functions. It causes you to slow down long enough to allow your brain to catch up.

Writing something with your own hand makes it more permanent. There's no backspace, no delete key. It's more serious, more meaningful. Writing your intentions – your promises to yourself for health and fitness change, and to finally go after your most important goals – allows your unconscious mind to believe you more than if you tap them into an app that can be deleted. And that meaning and trust cements your intentions enough to allow them to become habit.

> *All the data gathered suggest that the difference between the 20% and the 80% can be reduced to one thing: Habit.*

Beyond the neuroscience and the other unseen mumbo-jumbo, there are practical reasons that a physical planner of this sort is preferable to a digital app. You can take it into the gym without worrying about dropping it, crushing it, or dripping sweat all into its sensitive components to muck up the works. You can easily jot notes with pen without having to power up, bypass security protocols, and scroll through several screens in search of the right icon.

Sometimes old school really is the best school.

We chose to integrate nutrition and fitness into your daily planner for much of the same reasons that it is necessary to integrate them into your daily life. We want you to succeed at your health and fitness. We also want you to accomplish the big things you've always wanted. And we know that you need to take steps every day toward success. This planner will help you do that.

In this planner you can record how much water you drank during your three-hour meeting while still in the meeting. You can plan workouts into your upcoming business travel because they're both on the same page. You will be cued to make sure you have a healthy brown bag lunch on Tuesday for the four-hour strategy session at work because you are planning your meals on the same page that you have scheduled the meeting. You'll be able to decrease the space between you and your long-term goals because you'll see and schedule the daily steps you need to take to get there. By integrating your nutrition and fitness planning into your daily planner, you more readily make it a habitual part of your daily life.

Why four weeks?

This workbook is intended to inform your fitness and weight loss efforts with the latest science in nutrition and wellness, so that all the pieces in this weight-loss puzzle finally come together. The System is designed to help you create a solid framework for a new, complete wellness lifestyle.

Planners tend to come in six-month, 12-month, even 18-month increments. Fitness and weight-loss plans tend to come in 12-week denominations. Why four weeks?

Four weeks – 28 days – is a bite-sized bit, in which you can intently focus on doing the activities you'll be learning, that you wish to make habitual parts of your regular lifestyle. While much was made previously of the 21-day period needed to make new habits, behavioral psychology research has turned that number on its head. In fact, big changes can take more like 66 days on average to become automatic, and possibly longer.[3]

Many fitness plans that are big undertakings – aptly called "challenges" – tend to run 12 weeks, or 90 days. That period may encompass the 66-day mark, but it can be daunting to many. It's long enough to naturally divide itself into three parts – beginning, middle, and end – allowing for a period of burn-out, for a time of rationalized "cheating" or "backsliding."

It's easier to convince yourself that you're too busy, or the time wasn't right, to commit to a 12-week challenge. And then it allows for disappointment that your results weren't as dramatic as you expected at the end of your long, hard-working 12 weeks (because you've already forgotten about the cheat and its consequences.)

Just four weeks is long enough for you to make significant changes in your behavior, to encourage you that it's possible, and to produce enough physical changes to keep you motivated to continue until the behavior becomes an automatic HABIT.

Take a week (we call it Week 0) to work through the workbook and goal-setting exercises, and then see what you can accomplish with focused effort, once all the pieces of the puzzle are in place, in four weeks! It's easy – and powerful – to divide your efforts into four-week increments so that you have a natural mental break, even when you continue your new success behaviors (with the Healthy Habits System™ 90-Day Planner) without skipping a beat.

Four-week cycles allow you a natural cadence for data collection so that you can give your solid efforts to behaviors for four weeks, but if your body seems to stop responding, you can troubleshoot your efforts at the beginning of a new four-week cycle.

We have intentionally developed the planner system so that you can continue using it to track all aspects of your abundant life. Once you have fully attained your goals, after the dust settles from the celebration that you'll have duly and rightfully earned, you can continue in your habits with the benefit of the Healthy Habits System™ 90-Day Planner.

Let your habits integrate into your day, and watch the pieces fall together, allowing you to finally maintain your transformation. If one day you find your pants fitting tighter, the System allows for periodic four-week cycles to rework the workbook, re-focus intently, and recalibrate your routines to guard against the slippage that causes weight regain.

HABITS lead. RESULTS follow.

Where your habits lead you – to health and fitness success, or to increasingly serious health challenges – depends solely on the type of habits you practice. The beautiful thing about habits is that the bad ones can be broken and replaced with new, good habits.

Habits are not static, nor are they set in stone. You really can change your direction by changing your habits. You are not stuck, nor are you fated for poor health. Scientific studies of ever-increasing sophistication are showing that even the most disadvantageous genetic profiles are overcome by healthy habits. You are not destined to experience all the health challenges your parents did. Your lifestyle matters much more than the genes you've inherited. You. Are. In. Control.

Yet you may not feel as though you are. That is likely because you have unknowingly developed bad habits. It's a rare person, indeed, that wakes up one morning and firmly decides, "Today, I am going to start killing myself with bad choices." Instead, we generally stumble into our habits accidentally, and usually because we're busy or distracted by all the many other things vying for our attention.

Other habits are a result of our upbringing, or misinformation, or even lack of information. We simply don't know what we don't know, until a medical crisis surprises us with the lesson. By that time, while our resolve to change is strongly motivated, we have a lot of un-learning to do and that can be intimidating, even overwhelming. We've developed tastes for unhealthy foods and aversions to healthy ones. We've built harried, frazzled schedules without a lot of room for proper exercise or sleep. We've neglected simple things, like drinking enough water. We may not know what we don't know, but we know what we don't like! Unless we create a framework – a system – that allows us to love the thing we hate, and makes the hard thing easy to do, we are much more likely to continue in our bad habits, despite the fact that we know they are killing us.

Here's another surprise. What you think are good habits may be hurting you. Do you diet often? Do you demonize foods, labeling them as evil so that you'll stay away from them? Do you reduce your calories so much that you're too tired to exercise? These efforts can and do result in initial weight loss – and can lead to weight regain. Why? Because they are not sustainable. You can't make a permanent and positive habit out of restrictive diets – but you can unwittingly create a negative habit of yo-yo dieting, which will land you squarely in the 80%.

Another example. What do you do before you go to bed? Do you cram in a workout in the hours before sleep? Do you work on your computer in bed? Watch television until you fall asleep on the couch? Do you end your day with a nightcap, hoping for it to relax you into sleep?

These habits may actually keep you from restorative sleep, which impacts your health in complex ways and results in low energy, poor memory and cognitive function – and weight gain.

Constant sleep deprivation makes you crave sugars for quick energy while reducing your metabolic rate and ability to burn the added sugar. Regular sleep restriction creates a cortisol environment that primes you for Type 2 diabetes, and keeps you locked in the 80%. The Healthy Habits System™ was created to serve as a framework you can use to pinpoint the harmful habits you have unknowingly developed, and intentionally create healthy habits to take their place.

The Healthy Habits System™ Workbook is your guide through habit planning, and the 90-Day Planner facilitates their practice. The System integrates four aspects of a healthy lifestyle – how you eat, drink, move, and sleep – with your daily scheduling and planning needs, so that you can begin visualizing how these habits can become rituals in your daily life and save you from the neglect that so often afflicts high-achieving individuals. It brings your long-term goals and dreams closer by empowering you to create daily steps toward them. The Healthy Habits System™ recognizes that you have one life and is here to help you make every day of it count.

The Healthy Habits System™ will prove to you that you can succeed in your career, your family, your education, and your fitness – all at the same time. All you need is a framework that makes doing the right things easier than not.

You CAN join the 20%. You CAN create a lifestyle you enjoy that safeguards your health and fitness, that lets you turn your health around, and lets you permanently disembark the weight-loss roller coaster. Not only are you in charge, *you deserve to be*. You are worth it.

You are worthy of the effort and the freedom it will bring. No more negative, harmful habits.

It's time to say YES!

PART 1: DO

Planful Living Strategies to Meet All Your Goals

DO IS THE FIRST section of the workbook because its information is crucial to applying the Healthy Habits System™. You will be inspired as you read it to take on many of your long-held dreams and goals, outside of weight loss and fitness, by breaking them down into doable chunks. With these principles, you can finally see them come to pass in your life! The DO sections of Educate, Evaluate, and Create are all together so you can sail through this topic and use its insights as you go through the rest of the workbook.

CHAPTER 1: EDUCATE

How to use your time planfully.

*Before you start moving a bunch of stuff, make a plan so you know
you have a place to put it all.*
- Paul L. Waldrop, Sr.

U NLESS YOU ALREADY have the life you want, in its entirety, then there's something uncomfortable you need to know: You can't have the life you want, and the life you have now, at the same time.

Some things about the life you HAVE will necessarily need to change or evolve so that you can have the life you WANT.

It may seem pretty obvious, but the things you are doing every day need to be in support of your long-term goals and dreams. Things you do that are not helping you make progress toward what's important are probably detracting from those instead. Very few things you do with your time are impact-neutral on your dreams. Except for things like brushing your teeth, an action is not impact-neutral. It is either advancing you or is a waste of time.

So, how do you spend your time? There are 24 hours in a day, and seven days in a week. That's 168 hours that each person has, each week. Rich or poor, busy or bored, we all have the same amount of time to spend or waste at our pleasure. While you can always make more money, you can never make more time. Once it's gone, you can't get it back. Money comes and goes, but time just – goes. So, how you planfully use it is important.

These things said, it's important to have downtime. You can't be effective over the long-term if you're trying to make, drive, create or accomplish something during all your waking hours. If you try burning the candle at both ends for too long, your journey won't be as enjoyable, either. You need to be able to work hard, move fast and post gains on whatever scoreboard is important to you. You also need to be able to look back and see the whole-life value your journey has represented. Stay balanced and you'll be more likely to live a happy life.

CHAPTER 2: EVALUATE

Where is your time spent now?

Dost thou love life? Then do not squander time, for that is the stuff life is made of.
- Benjamin Franklin

THINK BACK OVER the last two weeks and list the things that take the most of your time. Don't get too detailed, but do really think about it. Don't just list, "Doing my job," as one of the items. What specific element of your job takes time to do?

List things like sleep and exercise, preparing food, as well as family time such as spending time with the kids, going to church or civic volunteer work, etc. How do you see yourself spending time right now? Spend five minutes listing how you spend your 168 hours per week.

You may use the Activity table in your worksheet package, or simply make your own: Draw a grid with two columns – labeled "Activity" and "Hours Spent per Week" – and however many rows you need. (Some people prefer to do a multi-week time log where they can get an accurate view of time spent. That's a worthwhile exercise, but will take you some time. For the purposes of this workbook, just populate this the best you can. If you do a detailed time study, come back and revise this section.)

Now, list your most important dreams and goals for your life in the downloadable worksheet. You can revisit this later, and you should from time to time. For now, write down a few major things you want to do in your life, and write at least one thing you want to accomplish or see happen this year, and if you can, write one for this month, and one for this week.

Next, look at both lists together *without judgment*. Many people find that they have been spending at least some time doing things they know are not associated with a dream or big goal they have. This means one of two things: 1) You have a goal or dream you forgot to write about, but that you regularly spend time working toward, or 2) You have let idle time get taken by unimportant things that you don't truly desire to do.

Don't worry about having to move things from one answer to the other, and don't feel bad if, for example, you forgot to write family-oriented things on your list of dreams and needed your time log to tell you what's important. We all get busy. Just go revise your goals/dreams to include the things you forgot.

For the things that you can't add to your goals/dreams list because you don't believe they are important, actively begin to discover ways to free up that time so you can spend it on things you do dream of. Be mindful that this may be a process. If you're in a job that doesn't advance your dreams, you may have life responsibilities that mean you can't simply quit tomorrow and go get a new one. Embrace the process and learn from it. But do embrace it.

Effort/Desire Misalignment will lead to frustration and even depression, and you certainly don't have time for that.

CHAPTER 3: CREATE

Plan to make your dreams come true

A goal without a plan is just a wish.
- Antoine de Saint-Exupéry

Now that you have an idea of how you spend your time, and how well that aligns to your truest desires and dreams, you're ready to move to the next phase. With your long-term dreams in mind, what is a big goal you want to achieve this year? Do you have more than one? Can you realistically get them all done in one year?

As you plan each day, keep your short-, medium- and long-term goals in mind. You'll also learn more about creating short-, medium-, and long-term fitness goals and how they can motivate your daily activities (and feed your progress toward your life goals!) in the Move sections coming up.

There are mundane things that you will no doubt need to do each day, but be sure you are making progress toward something you truly desire. Don't forget to enjoy the journey – just be sure it's a journey that's leading somewhere.

A note about focus:

Be mindful of the day and the future as they are one in your life. You can't separate future from present, since what you do today determines a lot about tomorrow. However, you CAN be present in today, and you CAN'T be present in the future (or the past). You can't interact with those times directly. If you keep your mind on the future too much, you'll miss important experiences that happen in the present, and your future will be spent wishing you had enjoyed the journey more. Don't do that. Enjoy the trip. Just be sure it's a trip that goes somewhere. Don't get to the end and realize you hadn't used every opportunity to enjoy this life.

Hunter S. Thompson said it well: "Life should not be a journey to the grave with the intention of arriving safely in a pretty and well-preserved body, but rather to skid broadside in a cloud of smoke, thoroughly used up, totally worn out, and loudly proclaiming "Wow! What a ride!" (Hunter S. Thompson, The Proud Highway: Saga of a Desperate Southern Gentleman, 1955–1967) You may prefer a milder sentiment, but the point is that we should live each day to its fullest, yet find a way to set up the next day to be even better, and draw even closer to our goals.

Basics:

As you plan each day, a few things are important to do:

Have a Block Schedule. If you use Outlook or another similar day management tool, then you are already familiar with block scheduling. There is a Block Schedule in your planner to use for things that need to happen at a certain time. Leave space between things that are scheduled far apart during your day so that you can write in things that come up. When you have big open spots, that's where you can work on your Task List. The block schedule in your planner is intentionally not pre-populated with times for each block. Everybody plans and does their day differently. Rather than waste space writing in prescribed times where you may not do any pre-planned work, we've left room for you to organize the day YOU have.

Time	Activity

This is an example of the Block Schedule provided in the Daily Spread.

Your Task List: It's true that nothing happens at all that doesn't happen at a certain time, but not everything needs its timeslot predetermined. Keep a Master Task List (you'll find one in your 4-Week Planner) of things you need to do, and take the ones that specifically need to be done each day and write them down on that day's page.

If it's on your mind, write it down. As you come up (as we all do) with what can seem to be an endless supply of new things to do, write them on your Master Task List. Even insignificant things can eat at your attention until you write them down, so observe this principle always: "If it's on your mind, write it down." Get it out of your head. Humans have a limited capacity for the number of unique things we can keep attention on at the same time, and if you have 6 or 7 "to do" items running around in your head, you likely won't have too many new, innovative ideas. Not convinced? Try it for a week. Write down new tasks as they come to you, and believe that they will still be written there when you do your daily planning. Forget about them until then. See if you don't become more creative, productive, energetic and happy.

Today's Tasks	Big Three U x I = T

This is an example of the Daily Task List provided in the Daily Spread.

Score your Big Three according to the Urgency and Importance Scale, discussed next, each day.

Evening Ritual: Each evening, review the day you just had and see what got done and what remains to be done. Write things you'll do the next day on that day's list. Things that fell off because they were unimportant go back on the Master Task List. Don't do something just because it's on your Master Task List.

Sometimes we start thinking of a million things to do and we'll write many of them down. But later it becomes apparent that those things aren't associated with a long-term goal, and so get deleted or delegated. Be willing to let go of things you realize you don't need.

The Big Three: Once you have reclaimed meaningful undone things from the day, write down any additional things you need to for the next day.

When you have your Task List, go through and pick the Big Three. These are the three things that you really need to get done, even if the rest of your schedule gets derailed. Some days you may only have one thing.

A lot of people have trouble with the Big Three exercise, so don't worry if that's you. In fact, most start the exercise believing they aren't having trouble, just that they have 20 things to do that are all the most important. If that's you, try this method:

Urgency x Importance --> Big Three
U x I = T

1. Assign an *Urgency (U)* ranking to each item, ranked 1 to 3. "1" means that the impact of this not getting done will be felt immediately in a measurable way. "3" would mean that it's either a distant future impact or not a big problem if it goes undone.

2. Assign an *Importance (I)* ranking to each item, ranked 1 to 3. "1" means this is very high in terms of dollar cost, reputation impact, impact on other costly project elements, etc. As before, "3" denotes little importance.

3. Multiply the Urgency and Importance scores and record the *Totals (T)*. The lowest overall scores are your Big Three. (You usually won't have more than three). Circle the lowest three scores, and do those items first.

Here are a few examples:

• Make the house payment, due in 30 days.

This one would score a 1 on Importance, but a 3 on Urgency. It's going to be a big deal if you don't do it, but it's not due for 30 days, so it can wait.

• Make the house payment, due today.

This would still score a 1 on importance, but is now a 1 on Urgency also. If you don't pay it today, you may get a late fee and impact your credit score.

• Put out a fire in the oven.

This is a 1 and 1, and if we were ranking all 3 of these together, paying the house payment would now be a 2. There won't be a house to pay for if it burns down. So, as you see, scores are relative to one another.

Then, fill out your block schedule showing how and when you will do each major thing, making sure to allocate enough time to do the Big Three.

Here's a trick: If you have an item on your list that's either hard to do or requires a lot of concentration, schedule it first. Early in the morning is when you have the most energy, and is also when others are (in many businesses) less likely to interrupt you. Your particular circumstance may differ, but studies do show that our ability to sustain focus on difficult tasks is higher in the morning than later in the day. You're more likely to decide late in the day that the hard Big Three item can wait until tomorrow, but that just makes it more likely to be a high urgency item once you finally get to it. You'll more likely do it today if you do it early.

Schedule things that require more talking and social interaction for later in the day. Also, don't be surprised if your rhythm changes over time. You may find in your 20s that you do a lot of great work after 5 PM when everyone else goes home, and in your 40s and 50s you may switch to getting your best work done between 7 AM and 8 AM before anyone else is in the office. Stay in tune with your body and mind and maximize your effectiveness by working with, not against them.

Wrapping it Up: So, you've got your master task list, your daily task list, your big 3 and your block schedule. Now, as you move through your day, feel free to adjust as you go to maximize your effectiveness. Each evening, be sure to look at the day ahead. Don't do this in bed. Get this finished at least an hour before bedtime. This will give you time to wind down and not think about work in a way that interrupts your sleep. (See the workbook section on Sleep for more information on this.)

Start each day with a plan already in-hand, and you'll be approximately 1.5 to 2.5 hours ahead of most of the rest of the population. You'll get more accomplished and get closer to your goals. This will literally give you up to 12.5 hours more effective time to work on your dreams than the average person gets in a typical workweek. If you take two weeks' vacation (so you work 50 weeks per year), then that's another 625 hours you'll spend achieving your dreams each year. It's the equivalent of hiring a part time worker to achieve your dreams for you!

You can't manufacture more time each week, but you can spend your 168 hours the way the highest achieving people do, and realize that to be in the top 1% of achievers, all it takes is a little planning and a lot of discipline.

Do this every single day.

As you go through your day using your planner, use the Healthy Habits System™ elements of Eat, Drink, Move and Sleep to log and plan your meals, workouts, hydration and sleep strategy.

About the Master Task List:

You've been writing things on your Master Task List that came to you so that you could get them out of your head and use your brain capacity for creative thoughts. Once per week, go to that list and keep it healthy. Trim it like an arborist would trim a grove of trees. In order to keep the arbor healthy, the pruner needs to come and take off little branches that don't fit the design.

In the same way, you need to take out of your list things that you thought you needed to do, but that don't align your effort (that it would take to do them) with something that's on your dream list, or your list of short-, medium- or long-term goals. You must be ruthless about this in order to protect your dreams. Delegation: If it's something that has to be done, but not necessarily by you, find a way to hire it done or delegate it. If you have to be the one to do it, find the time and get it off of your list, or delete it and be ok with it not getting done.

Rituals and Habits: You need to create rituals and habits in your life. Things you do every day or every week pretty much the same way can be done with minimal creative effort. This leaves more room for you to innovate and advance your goals. Don't let your life become mundane – that's not what we're suggesting. Simply make a system out of what you can so that what can't be systematized can emerge as the fulfilling, adventurous, full-engagement activity that it should be.

Do you cook every day? If that's what you truly enjoy, then keep doing it. If you think of it as a necessary chore (one of those mundane things mentioned earlier), then start pre-cooking and take back that time. Do you spend half of every Summer Saturday mowing the lawn? If you enjoy that, fine! If not, there is likely a young person with a lawnmower in your neighborhood who is eager to start a business. Help your neighbor out and get back that time to be with your family and achieve your dreams.

Do you want to start a business? How much time per week would that take? We just showed you how you can have an additional 12.5 hours of productivity. Could you take some of that back in the afternoons or early evenings and work on your project? Could you use those Saturday hours? What about the hours you spend cooking on weeknights? Could you microwave delicious, nutritious things you precooked and use the time you get back to visit with your family? (If you have a family and you're starting a business or working on a big project for a company, you need every chance you can get to spend time with them.)

Use the Healthy Habits System™, along with these Planful-Living Strategies, to transform your life and put your 168 hours to use making big, fun-filled strides toward your dreams.

PART 2: EDUCATE

Learn the System

CHAPTER 1: EAT

Nutrition best practices for successful meal planning and portion control.

Great things are done by a series of small things brought together.
- Vincent van Gogh

WE ARE OBSESSED with finding The Right Eating Plan, which can be translated two ways: "the best way to eat the most without gaining weight," or, "the easiest way to lose weight without really trying."

Plans are a great place to start, especially if the plan in question provides sufficient nutrients in proper proportions. Plans provide a framework; obviously, we love frameworks. They provide guidelines for self-discovery. And that's a good thing. It's vitally important that you discover what foods work best for you, which foods you love and which you can learn to love, and which foods cause you distress (ie, allergies and/or sensitivities). But what happens when you stop doing the plan?

There are a couple of basic truths you need to understand about all plans:

1. They all work while you are working them. There is not one single plan that is optimal for everyone, nor is there one plan that works better than another. The plan doesn't work – YOU work the plan.

2. Unless you can make it habit – in other words, you love the food and method of eating, and it fits your life easily – you will not maintain your results. Period. End of story.

In other words, there is no such thing as The Right Eating Plan. At the end of the day, plans are trumped by Best Nutrition Practices.

Side note: Fad diets should be avoided. For the record, "fad diet" can be defined as any dietary framework that
1. Eliminates entire food groups or decreases macronutrient intake substantially and dangerously below recommended daily intakes (RDI);
2. claims rapid weight loss (more than 2lbs/week) without the discomfort of hunger; or
3. relies on juices, shakes, or food products more than on real, whole foods.

Fad diets are never meant to fit a healthy lifestyle. Fad diets are not sustainable.

So then, what are Nutrition Best Practices?

Eat fresh, natural foods.

Eat vegetables in abundance. Consume low-glycemic fruit daily. Add a serving of protein to every meal to increase satiety and to support muscle mass during a caloric deficit. Do not neglect starch and other carbohydrate foods as they are your body's preferred energy source. To illustrate this fact, nutrition scientists are fond of saying, "fat is burned in a furnace of carbohydrate." If you have a gluten/grain intolerance make sure you're consuming enough starchy vegetables to replace grains. Eat a variety of foods to make sure you get all the vitamins and minerals necessary for proper function.

Eat fat.

Healthy fats are a vital component of your physiology. They make up the membranes of your cells. Your brain is about 60% fat in structure. There are some fats that you must eat because you can't make them—they are the essential omega-3 (N-3) and omega-6 (N-6) fatty acids. If you don't eat fatty fish regularly and you do eat processed foods, your diet provides an overabundance of N-6 fats and a deficiency of N-3 fats, which can lead to inflammatory conditions that allow disease to thrive. Find a good fish oil supplement and take it daily.[iv]

Eat salmon and other wild-caught, cold water fish weekly. Other good fat sources are extra virgin olive oil, avocado oil, coconut oil (in moderation), avocados, nuts and seeds and butters made from them (in moderation), coconut milk, and olives. Fat is more calorically dense than any of the other macronutrients, so you don't need as much of it, but do not make the mistake of eliminating it. Aside from fish oil, other animal fats are generally correlated with cardiovascular disease, so it's best to consume lean and low-fat animal products, and rely on plants for your fats.

Avoid added sugars.

If you want to "cut carbs" look to added sugars. If you eliminate any food, eliminate sugary processed foods. Sugar-sweetened beverages, baked goods, candies, and even savory processed foods contain added sugar. The typical fruity yogurt sold in the United States contains more sugar than a serving of ice cream. Let that sink in. Something you probably thought was good for you is actually worse than something you thought was bad for you. With that in mind…

Refuse to label foods as "good" or "bad".

Food is food – inanimate, amoral, objective. Foods are neither good or bad in and of themselves. Some ingredients are better consumed only moderately or in small amounts while others should be ingested liberally.

Labeling foods as good or bad inevitably leads to disordered eating. Although, you need to understand the difference, as far as the Healthy Habits System™ is concerned, between "foods" and "food products." A variety of real, whole, unprocessed foods should be enjoyed several times each day, but processed food products should be limited in a healthy diet. You will find it much easier to avoid processed sugars, added preservatives and excess sodium, chemical additives, and unhealthy fats if you limit your intake of processed foods.

Whole foods include: fresh fruits and vegetables, as well frozen fruits and veggies without additives; fresh meats, whole grains (brown and wild rice, quinoa, old fashioned and steel-cut oats, etc.), sprouted grain breads and baked products, nuts and no-additive nut butters, and unflavored dairy products.

A good rule of thumb is that you generally find whole foods along the perimeter of your grocery store, and that is where you should spend most of your grocery budget. Processed foods include premade meals, frozen dinners, frozen vegetables with sauces, canned fruits and vegetables, instant grain products (minute rice, quick-cooking and instant oatmeal, etc.) breakfast cereals, baked goods, chips, etc.

Now, all the previous points together have likely been easier to read than this next one. Read it anyway…

There's no such thing as a free lunch – or free calories.
If you consume more than you burn, you will gain weight. Regardless of how "clean" and healthy your diet is, everyone is still subject to the laws of thermodynamics. That is not said to simplify the whole kettle of fish with what has become, to some, the emotionally-charged statement, "calories in vs calories out."

There are lots of individual differences that impact the rate of caloric burn, causing one person to burn calories at a lower or higher rate than another. But still, you can't expect to consume an unlimited amount of energy and not have to either burn it or store it, even if the source of that energy is organic and minimally processed.

It's important enough to say again – there is no free lunch, and there is no escaping our need to moderate our consumption. However, if the idea of counting calories is a deal-breaker for you, either due to boredom or busy schedule – good! Counting calories is too time-intensive and restrictive to be a sustainable behavior. The superior nutrition best practice is to observe portion control instead. Find a visual representation that best approximates your proper portion for any food, and ensure you remain relatively true to that eyeball evaluation.

Meal Planning & Prepping for Maintenance Success

There can often be what feels like an unpassable chasm between knowing and doing. That principle is proven out, time and again, in weight loss efforts. It can also be what makes the difference between weight loss maintenance and reversion.

As we discussed, there are strategies for success that the 20% have effectively incorporated into their daily lives that enable them to maintain their weight loss. Successful maintainers have learned that the best way to permanently cross the chasm between knowing and doing is to make doing the only option. When you habitually remove failure from the equation, the only outcome is success.

Two crucial habits that practically guarantee weight loss and maintenance success are meal planning and pre-cooking. Budget-minded cooks have used meal planning strategies for generations. In some respects, however, it's a lost art as so many domestic skills are not as widely taught as they had previously been.

You may already use a grocery list to guide your shopping (and you can find a list template in your worksheet package and for download at https://www.clearpathfitness.com/healthy-habits-system-free-download). Meal planning takes that organizational strategy a step further by guiding what you put on your list and using everything you buy. It's a way to make sure you stick to your meal plan by having the foods you need on hand. But it's incomplete by itself.

You can make a meal plan and a shopping list as carefully as possible, and buy only what's on the list, but failure is still an option if you get swept away in the whirlwind of activity we call LIFE and don't have time to make your meals. This is a big reason why prepared foods have become such big business in the diet industry. Pre-packaged foods are convenient – eliminating planning, effort, and choices, making success the most probable outcome for dieters.

Nonetheless, it's unsustainable. Nobody can live on a prepackaged meal plan forever. They are expensive, they lack adequate variety, and they are targeted in their caloric and nutrient construction for weight loss, not weight maintenance. Unless you learn how to plan, portion, and prepare your own healthy meals, you will find it extremely difficult to maintain weight loss achieved through a prepackaged foods diet system.

The thing that makes meal planning and careful shopping a complete strategy – as well as a sustainable and economical alternative to prepackaged diets – is prepping your meals in advance, or pre-cooking. It's a strategy that bodybuilders and physique athletes have used for years. And it's now a vital tool in your Healthy Habits™ toolbox.

Each week through this 28-day journey includes a weekly planning spread complete with an EAT Weekly Menu Template, which is part of your download package. Plan meals – breakfasts, lunches, dinners, and snacks – and write them in their respective grids. Plan leftovers from dinner Monday night for lunch Tuesday (for example). Plan snacks that can be easily packed, carried, and repeated throughout the week.

Carry healthy snacks with you in your backpack, purse, briefcase or car, so you're never without a healthy choice when hunger strikes away from home. Most importantly, plan meals that you can make in advance, so that packing it for work or putting it on the table after work is so simple that fast food would be an inconvenience.

It is always more efficient to prepare several meals in one four-hour event than it is to prepare one meal in a 30- or 45-minute kitchen event. Think about it: each time you cook, you must also clean, thus making the short kitchen session more like 60–90 minutes for one meal. Doing that only once every day adds up to more than 10 hours a week!

Instead, you could combine pre-cooking four or five large dishes that can be portioned into multiple servings and meals, into one kitchen event, with only one dishwashing episode. You can easily reduce that 10+ hour commitment by half each week. Not bad!

Everything you need is washed, perfectly portioned, and ready to grab when you're packing up for the day, thus saving you time in the mornings without relying on meals out. No more fast food lunches for you, when you have delicious homecooked meals on the ready. No more foraging for snacks when you're distracted by pressing tasks and to-do lists. No more decision fatigue, because you already know what to eat! And (bonus) no more food waste and broken food budgets!

If you are new to advanced meal prepping, plan for some added expense on the front end, as you will need to stock up on packaging items, foods, and perhaps cooking supplies. With that in mind, *plan your Week 0 for the beginning of a pay period, and budget accordingly.* The initial meal prep session may be a bit intimidating if you are unaccustomed to assembly-line cooking, but it will become a time-saving habit, and you'll be amazed at how easy it makes sticking to your healthy eating plan.

Your goal with the Healthy Habits System™ Planners is to create healthy habits you can easily continue doing for the rest of your life, so you become one of the successful transformation maintainers. When you've completed your four weeks with the Planner, you'll continue planning your meals and pre-prepping food so that continued success is the only possible outcome.

Following are some meal-prep tips that can help you save time from the moment you get home from the store, and may even trigger some new ideas of your own.

Meal prep tips

Fruit

- Buy in season – fresher, more nutrient-rich, cheaper
- Wash hard fruits; place in a bowl where you can see it, so it's easy to get to.
- Wash all berries right before eating/packing for the day for optimal freshness and longevity.
- Portion and thaw frozen fruits.
- Cut and cube melons, package in portions.

Vegetables

- Buy in season – fresher, more nutrient-rich, cheaper
- Wash when you get home with your bounty.
- Cut hard vegetables and portion into Ziploc baggies with nuts for easy-access snacks.
- Tear lettuces, cut cabbage; store in large Ziploc bags or sealable bowls with a paper towel.
- Roast or sauté (squashes, greens, cruciferous) using high-heat oils, broths, and vinegars. Store with protein and starch for meals on the go.

Crockpot meals

- Choose recipes with ingredients found on The List
- Always make double/triple recipes. Leftovers can be lunches for the week, or frozen for up to three months.
- Package leftovers in individual portions for faster reheating and to avoid waste.
- Leftovers are safe to eat when stored in airtight containers refrigerated for 3–5 days, and in the freezer for three months.

Oven meals
- Choose recipes that use ingredients on The List.
- Always make double/triple recipes. Leftovers can be lunches for the week, or frozen for up to three months.
- Package leftovers in individual portions for faster reheating and to avoid waste.

Miscellaneous
- Build an inventory of airtight containers and Ziploc baggies of various sizes.
- Stock up on meats when on sale, and plan one large meal prep session to stock your freezer
- at the beginning of your pay period.
- Label everything (food name and date) before freezing.

CHAPTER 2: DRINK

Hydration strategies for weight loss and maintenance

Thousands have lived without love, not one without water.
- W. H. Auden

PROPER HYDRATION IS AS IMPORTANT to the Healthy Habits System™ as what you eat, how well you sleep, and how much you move. Your body's healthy functioning is dependent on water. Every metabolic process uses water. Brain function requires sufficient hydration. Proper blood pressure maintenance involves ample hydration.

Despite how important proper hydration is to optimal health and fitness, most people – even those that are highly conscious of eating properly and exercising regularly – don't have a strategy to ensure that they drink enough water to support their bodies. That can be a success-hampering mistake. Your body needs water, and when you are habitually dehydrated (as most are), it will send you signals to get you to drink water. That is thirst. The thing is, you are already dehydrated and need to catch up by the time you recognize that you are thirsty. If you ignore the thirst signal, or choose a non-hydrating beverage instead (such as soda or iced tea) your body will send a hunger signal. That's because you can harvest water from many foods.

Further, you may find it surprising that your body retains water, giving you that bloated, puffy look, when you don't drink enough of it. That's because it is such a necessary component of your vital systems that your physiology will do everything it can to protect you from losing too much. If, however, you drink enough water to support your systems, water retention will decrease. To avoid dehydration, as well as the water retention and possible overeating that could come from it, form habits that help you stay hydrated.

Let's look at a few suggested habits to ensure you stay hydrated:

- Buy a large insulated, dishwasher-safe, and leakproof water bottle that is comfortable to hold, carry, and drink from. Get one that won't embarrass you, because you'll be carrying it with you wherever you go. If you're motivated by pretty things, then go for it. If funky describes your eclectic fashion sense, then by all means – express yourself! Your water bottle will become a part of your daily ensemble (just like this planner, if you're using it right) so make sure you love it!
- Depending on the size of the bottle, you'll need to refill it repeatedly. Create a system to track how many bottles full of water you've had each day.
    - Refill it every time you go to the restroom.
    - Refill it at snacks and meals.
    - Wrap rubber bands around the base (or neck) and move them each time you empty it.
    - Use a dry erase marker to record hash marks each time you empty it; wipe them off at the end of the day to start fresh in the morning.
    - Drink water before, during, and after exercise. Empty your bottle at least one time during your workout. The more you sweat, the more you need.

You'll learn how to specifically calculate how much water you need to stay hydrated, regardless of your circumstances, in CREATE: DRINK.

A few words regarding water and other beverages. Many are not in the habit of drinking enough water because they drink other beverages throughout the day, that often add calories in the form of added sugars. Many dietitians and nutritionists argue emphatically that sugar-sweetened beverages are a root cause of the obesity epidemic – and they are not wrong. We are in the habit of reaching for beverages other than water to quench our thirst. In 2016, close to one-third of US adults consumed at least one sugar-sweetened beverage a day, presumably instead of plain water.

Drinking calorie-dense beverages, such as soda and fruit juices, has the unfortunate consequence of increasing your caloric intake without decreasing your hunger or your thirst. Add to that equation the fact that many sodas are also caffeinated, therefore dehydrating, (which, as previously discussed, can lead to overeating) it can be safe to assume that they have no regular place in a healthy lifestyle. In fact, many have reported significant weight loss by merely cutting out daily sodas.

If you think that diet sodas are exempt, think again. They dehydrate you AND add to your chemical load, giving your metabolism a harmful 1–2 punch. Diet sodas should be eliminated completely. The Healthy Habits System™ omits sodas and other sugar-sweetened beverages from your daily plan. If you crave sodas during the week, add it to your cheat/treat meal, but even then, make sure you stay hydrated by adding eight ounces of water for your cheat beverage.

Saving sodas for your weekly treat make them a special item rather than a daily crutch. You decrease your overall caloric load, and you allow your body the proper hydration it deserves. You may find, as many before you have, that your palate adjusts to the refreshing quality of water, without the onslaught of cloying sugar-sweetened or artificially-sweetened beverages. Eventually, you may find that the cravings cease altogether.

Finally, a word on alcohol. There is some evidence that moderate consumption can safeguard against cardiovascular disease. You need to recognize, however, that alcohol contributes sugar and calories to your overall load. A ml of alcohol contributes 7 calories, to be exact.

Additionally, "moderate consumption" may be less than you realize. Researchers define it as ~1 serving/day for females, and ~2 servings/day for males. Habitually drinking more than that can lead to health detriments, especially in women; regular heavy consumption in women has been linked to breast and other types of epithelial cancers.

Finally, in addition to alcohol's caloric contribution and its dehydrating characteristics are your metabolism's order of operations. The liver will recognize alcohol as a toxin needing to be dealt with, and will prioritize it over fat burning. If your priority is to burn fat and lose weight, you may want to skip the daily glass of wine altogether to allow your body the chance to burn stored fat.

None of this is to say you must become a tea-totaller. Nor does it mean you should never again enjoy a soda. But when it comes to weight loss and maintenance, water should always be your beverage of choice, and all others should be moderated according to your goals.

CHAPTER 3: MOVE

Finding your workout muse and making movement a habit

He who would learn to fly one day must first learn to stand and walk and run and climb and dance; one cannot fly into flying.
- Nietzshe

YOUR BODY IS DESIGNED TO MOVE. The more time you spend in sedentary activity, regardless of the position, the more you increase your chances of health challenges. Moving your body encourages movement of the lymph, your body's built-in detoxification system.

Movement increases circulation, oxygen transport, and metabolic rate. Moving weight builds muscle mass and bone density, protecting your body from the atrophy that accompanies aging. Moving your body with speed and intensity increases your heart rate, blood flow, and caloric burn. But the only way you'll make movement a habit is if you love the movement, and you love the way it makes you feel. Otherwise it'll be a drudgery too easily abandoned, regardless of its health benefits.

The best way to make daily exercise HABIT is to absolutely love the exercise you are doing.

One of the key behaviors that has separated the 20% of successful weight maintainers from the 80% that have regained weight is *continued and consistent physical activity*. On average, successful weight maintainers exercise about an hour a day.

They spend at least seven hours a week engaged in physical activity – every week – for the rest of their lives. After five years, the odds of maintaining weight loss permanently are significantly increased. An hour of activity per day for five years is 1,825 hours. Might I suggest that the best way to guarantee that you'll spend that much time doing something, is to absolutely love the thing you are doing?

Make it your goal to discover activity you love doing so much that you couldn't imagine letting a day pass without getting your fix. That kind of activity is your workout muse. Obviously the Muse is an allegory, used in art to describe a compulsion to create. We use it in the Healthy Habits System™ to describe a compulsion to create peak physical fitness with activity you love.

The qualities of your workout muse.

She'll be beautiful, interesting, and fun to spend time with, yes. But your workout muse will also benefit you in more specific ways. There are three main aspects to holistic physical fitness, and your muse will help you address each of them in a way that is enjoyable, motivating, and downright fun to you.

Cardio. She will make your breath catch and your heart beat fast. She will help you burn fat while increasing your cardiovascular capacity. If you don't enjoy the monotony of a treadmill or other solitary gym machines, she will take you into a variety of group exercise classes or other activities. She will help you set goals that keep you interested in your training, and will excite you to wake up and train every day.

Strength training. She will make you stronger and better for spending time with her. She will help you build muscle mass and bone density, and by doing so, will help increase your metabolic rate. In this way, she will make your body more durable and your figure gravity-proof.

Functional fitness. She will make you more flexible, more agile, and able to do more even when she's not around. And while she will never push you beyond what your body is physically healthy enough to do today, she will help your body grow stronger by spending time with her. She will help you increase your flexibility, functional fitness, and endurance in such a way that your health will defy the ravages of age. She will make you better able to tackle everyday tasks while protecting you from imbalance and overuse injuries.

Making your muse your habit.

Regardless of how much you love doing the activity, regardless of how much better it makes you feel, you will not consistently do it if you haven't structured your schedule to not only accommodate it, but to make skipping out on it harder than not. Following are some strategies to ensure that you spend time with your muse on the regular, so that you can become a successful maintainer.

Make a standing date.

Don't just pencil your workouts in; schedule them in ink, with as much priority as any formal appointment with someone else. Use your Monthly Spread to plan your workout schedule for the month, and cross them off when you complete them. And protect these inked-in appointments with yourself. Don't let other things interfere with your sweat sessions.

Make it a standalone event.

Schedule your workouts during a time that nothing else can compete for your attention. If you have more energy and focus in the morning, before others in your house wake up, before work absorbs you and your energy, then work out in the morning. It's not surprising that so many high-achieving individuals work out first thing in the morning, as it enables easier focus on other tasks throughout the day. Wake up 30 minutes earlier each morning, even if you don't work out until later in the day, so that you have more time to get things done so they don't crowd into your scheduled workout time.

Make it easy to do.

Pack your gym bag or lay out your workout clothes before you go to bed at night. Leave a bottle of water waiting for you on the bathroom counter, with a sticky note reminding you to get your sweat on. Put your running shoes next to the door, complete with a fresh pair of socks to beckon you to run. Include a bottle of water and pre-workout snack in the gym bag. If you don't schedule it in the morning, structure your day so that your workout is during rush hour traffic. Going to the gym instead of sitting in traffic is a much better use of your time. Eliminate excuses with structure, so that when you feel tired, it will still be easier to work out than it will be to not.

Make it a social event.

Study after study has shown that the main thing that keeps successful maintainers committed to their workouts is working out with others. Community is crucial to your success. Humans need human interaction. And while some find solace in solitary exercise when their days immerse them in human interaction, others need a friendly connection to keep them committed to their fitness.

There are other ways to set yourself up for workout success. On a sheet of paper, take 5 minutes to list a few we missed.

The Healthy Habits System Optimal Fitness Strategy

The Healthy Habits System™ combines four components into the optimal fitness strategy: **Strength, Sweat, Flex,** and **Rest.** Each of these activities are necessary for holistic fitness. Your muscle, bones, and physiology need weight-bearing activity on the regular. Your heart and lungs require the sweaty work of cardiovascular training in order to continue functioning well. Your body and spirit need the agility and flexibility provided by restorative stretching, and your entire being must have a break occasionally to continue thriving. And while all successful fitness strategies will always have these four elements, the possible combinations are as limitless as those that employ them.

Strength

Strength training can be done with bodyweight, resistance bands, or weights. Bodyweight exercises are not only versatile, they are portable and can be done anywhere. Resistance bands are easy to pack and take along on business trips to make sure you get a muscle-pumping workout even when your hotel doesn't host a weight room.

Weight training encompasses a wide variety of disciplines and muscle sports, ranging from group exercise methodologies such as BodyPump and Crossfit to competitive sports such as powerlifting, strongman competitions and Olympic lifting. If the idea of repetitive-motion activities on a machine in the confines of a gleaming gym facility leaves you feeling empty inside, don't despair. There is always a muse for you that will help build your muscles. All it takes for you to find her is a willing curiosity and adventurous spirit. Whatever activities get you jacked, make sure you include Strength at least twice in your schedule, and you work all your muscle groups at least one time each week. An ideal beginner routine in the gym includes three workouts per week, alternating upper body and lower body focus.

CHIEF PLANNER TIP:

It's important to not only plan your strength workouts, but to record them as well. What exercises did you do? How much weight did you lift, and in how many reps? Planning is important so you make sure you strengthen all your muscle groups each week; record-keeping is important so you can continually build your strength by increasing your intensity and/or weight moved. You will find Strength Logs in the back of your planner. Take advantage of them!

Sweat

Sweat refers to cardiovascular training. Any activity that elevates your heartrate and pulse for at least 20–45 minutes per session. You can choose from so many options! Dancing, running, swimming, High-Intensity Interval Training (HIIT), a variety of martial arts practices, plyometrics, cycling, spinning, roller-blading, rowing, bootcamp, and any number of group fitness modalities that have been innovated over the years.

If Sweat for the sake of sweat makes you want to cry in despair and monotony, find an intriguing event that motivates you to sweat consistently so you can perform well. Beyond traditional running, cycling, and swimming events, there are obstacle course races in abundance and abounding independent and team adventure races.

If these events are cost prohibitive or require travel you are not in a position to take on, there are a variety of local sports and fitness clubs, from jogging and cycling to more organized sports like rowing, soccer and volleyball. Just like with Strength, there will be a Sweat muse for you! Include at least two Sweat sessions in your weekly schedule.

Flex

Flex can mean a five or 10-minute stretch session before or after your other workouts, or a formal yoga class. Anything that ensures your muscles and joints remain supple and flexible will protect you from overuse and imbalance injuries. Your weekly schedule should include one long Flex session (such as yoga) and five shorter sessions.

Rest

You may find it counterintuitive, but your body strengthens itself when you allow time for rest. Your workouts stimulate growth by causing microtears in your muscle tissue, and your rest periods allow them to heal and adapt so they can continue growing as your strength and endurance improve. Strenuous exercise is imperative for good health, but it is a stressor, physically and mentally. Keep in mind, though – not all stressors are bad! You need the balance between stress and rest to create an injury-proof level of fitness.

Make sure that you plan an active rest day on which your activities are restorative and destressing. Your yoga day (long Flex), for example, can be calming restorative yoga that stretches you and blisses you out simultaneously. Maybe you've always wanted to do Tai Chi in Central Park, or find long riverside hikes to be centering.

Whatever the case, make sure you take one or two days (depending on the intensity of the other activities in your fitness strategy) for active rest. And if you're completely tapped out from a week of crushing your Strength, Sweat, and Flex training, take a balancing day of complete and total Rest. Consider scheduling a massage or infrared sauna to coax your muscles into an even deeper restoration.

When and how much to move

Include the following in your Weekly Move Plan:

Strength:
- At least twice a week:
- Work each muscle group at least once
- Can organize into:
    - full-body circuits
    - opposing muscle groups
      (ex: chest and back, push and pull)
    - upper and lower body
    - complimentary muscle groups
      (ex: shoulders and chest, quads and glutes)

Sweat:
- Two to four times per week
- Incorporate cross-training – do a variety of Sweat activities.

Stretch:
- One long session (45 min-1 hr at least)
- Five short sessions
    - After Strength and Sweat warmups and workouts

Rest:
- Active rest – one or two days per week
- Complete rest – occasionally, as needed

CHAPTER 4: SLEEP

Prioritizing and maximizing sleep to enhance health and fitness

Sleep is the best meditation.
 - Dalai Lama

H OW LONG WE SPEND in sleep has drastically diminished over the past several decades. Americans reported sleeping an average of 8–10 hours nightly in the 1950s; by this past decade that number had decreased to less than seven hours. On top of that, a large percentage of us report poor sleep quality, so that even when we clock 7–9 hours of sleep we are still exhausted.

According to the National Healthy Sleep Awareness Project, at least 25 million adults suffered from obstructive sleep apnea in 2014.[v]

This destructive condition impairs sleep by blocking our ability to involuntarily inhale enough oxygen to stay asleep. It also degrades health by increasing risk of high blood pressure, heart disease, Type 2 diabetes, stroke, and depression, and quite possibly more.

We have yet to fully understand the entirety of sleep's restorative impact on our physiology. We've heard our entire lives that we should be getting eight hours of shut-eye a night. However, sleep *quality* is much more important that *quantity*. Your health, longevity, and effectiveness are benefited much more by six hours of fully restorative, apnea-free sleep than it is by nine hours of suboptimal sleep.

Sleep impacts every other area of the Healthy Habits System™. The importance of good restorative sleep to your overall health cannot be overstated (hence the bold type). Sleep deprivation has been documented to create a negative hormonal environment priming us for metabolic dysregulation. Without adequate sleep, your body actively resists weight loss by slowing down your metabolic rate as well as sending more hunger signals, specifically for easily-accessed sugars in highly-processed carbohydrate foods. So while your hormones are driving you to eat more sugar, they are also hampering your ability to burn them at peak efficiency, causing them to be stored as fat.

The hormonal impacts of sleep deficiency are near impossible to overcome by will power and exercise, so even if you are diligent in your dietary discipline and your early-morning cardio, fat loss will still be exceedingly difficult. Without adequate sleep, you'll be tempted to consume more caffeine to power through your day, setting you up for overconsumption and a subsequent bad night's sleep following.

Without adequate sleep, you won't be able to work out with peak efficiency and effort, especially in the morning. For those of us that have difficulty falling off and staying asleep, the good news is there are things we can do during the day and before bed that will make our time in bed both easier and more effective. Things as diverse as adequate sunlight exposure, proper nutrition, smart stimulant timing, workout scheduling, and strategic supplementation all impact your sleep. A good night's sleep truly starts in the morning.

Not surprisingly, insufficient sleep is more often caused by poor behaviors than by health conditions. We take our laptops to bed and work on emails or we watch late night television until we fall asleep. We allow our technology to distract us from a beneficial bedtime routine. Once we are adults and no longer have anyone to tell us to get ready for bed, we lack the psychological cues that make us sleepy. Instead, we spend too much time "cyberloafing" and not enough time resting.

It doesn't take long for this restricted sleep pattern to impact our productivity, and only slightly longer for it to damage our health. Again, poor habits have impacted our health, this time by impacting our sleep. And again – fortunately for us – poor habits can be replaced by good ones that can give us a boost to enhance our sleep and our health.

Following is a list of *Sleep Boosters* and *Sleep Disruptors. Sleep Boosters* are behaviors, food practices, and supplements that you can apply to overcome any obstacles preventing optimal sleep efficiency. Once you begin applying Sleep Boosters and learning which ones optimize your rest, you can create a bedtime routine that can rejuvenate you and literally change your life.

On the other hand, *Sleep Disruptors* are behaviors and food practices that impair our ability to get a good night's sleep, and should be avoided. If you have made any of these disruptors habits, you should go about breaking them and replacing them with Sleep Boosters.

You will create a bedtime routine by combining Sleep Boosters in the Create section of this workbook. As you are selecting Boosters to include in your routine, opt for behavior changes before you add supplements. If you are eating fresh foods from The List according to your dietary needs, you should be consuming adequate vitamins and minerals in your food, and risk overconsumption of certain nutrients if you blindly add supplements. The only exception to this is fish oil, as everyone should consume it daily. This is no small thing; certain nutrients can be problematic, not dissimilar from drugs, if overconsumed.

Sleep Booster Behaviors

- Get 30 minutes of sunlight exposure early in the day
- Curtail caffeine consumption before 2 pm
- Get regular exercise; stretch consistently
- Turn lights down 2–3 hours before bed
- Turn off all screened devices 1 hour before bed
- Consume a small, protein and low-glycemic carb snack before bed
- Practice a bedtime routine:
    - Wash – face, shower, bath
    - Dress – change into pjs or loungewear
    - Write – make a to-do list for the next day
    - Read – a paper book
    - Talk – have a real-life conversation
- Create the ideal sleep environment:
    - Cool – temperature range 62–68°
    - Dark – no blue light, blackout curtains
    - Quiet – excepting white noise and fans
    - Bare – sleep in minimal loose clothing
    - Sanctuary – Use bed only for sleeping, reading, talking, and lovemaking

- Sleep Booster Supplements
    - Vitamin D – up to 1000 IU at bedtime, if you are deficient[vi]
    - Magnesium – up to 250 mg at bedtime[vii]
    - Chamomile tea
    - Sleepytime™ Tea
    - Fish oil – 250 mg daily

Sleep Disruptor Behaviors – avoid:

- Consuming caffeine late in the day
- Eating a heavy dinner with too little fiber too late in the day
- Watching television until falling asleep
- Alcohol consumption too close to bedtime
- Cyberloafing on smart devices or personal computers
- Falling into bed without getting ready for bed
- Exercising <2 hours before bed
- Analgesic and antihistamine use too close to bed
- Midnight bedtime, even if rising after eight hours of sleep

PART 3: EVALUATE

*Mark Where You Are So You'll Know
How Far You Need to Go*

YOU ARE LIKELY more than eager to get started, but before you dive into your new lifestyle, spend a week with this Workbook. Week 0 is built in to the Workbook to keep the odds of failure and relapse minimal by allowing you to recognize what you're doing now that needs to change to allow for your success, and why.

Over the next three days, you will be recording as much data as possible regarding your current lifestyle, including what you eat and drink, your water intake, your current activity levels (including exercise, regular walking around, stretching, etc.), and how well you are sleeping. You will find samples of how to best use the Evaluate tracking pages following this section; the actual tracking pages are in your download package. We encourage you to fill them up with as much detailed, usable data you can.

From there, you will take the information you received in Educate and combine it with your data in Evaluate to Create your plan for the next four weeks. Finish up Week 0 by making preparations in Coordinate, so that you can hit the ground running in Week 1. (Refer back to your comprehensive <u>Healthy Habits System™ schedule.</u>)

CHAPTER 1: EAT AND DRINK

Three-day intake diary

The true secret of happiness lies in taking a genuine interest in all the details of daily life.
- William Morris

A T THE BEGINNING of a working relationship, dietitians and other health and wellness professionals have new clients document everything they eat and drink for three days, judgement free. This exercise accomplishes a couple of things: it gives the dietitian a glimpse into the client's food preferences and practices, AND it establishes a habit baseline. You already know your current preferences, but you may not be fully cognizant of your food habits.

In the first phase of your new healthy habit journey – what we call Week 0 – you'll complete a three-day Evaluation of your habits as they stand now, including a three-day intake diary in order to establish your own habit baseline. This will help you better understand what food habits – even (and especially) those you practice without thinking while you're occupied with the important things in your life – have brought you to your current fitness state. With this exercise, you'll begin to understand what habits you need to change in order to change your health. In your download package is a sample of a completed daily intake diary. Note that you will also record your water intake (Drink) at the bottom of this table. Again, this is not the place to create change. You will learn how much water you should drink daily to stay hydrated in EDUCATE: Drink.

You'll be recording everything you eat and drink for three days, including two weekdays and one weekend day. The goal is to record, not judge; don't change the way you eat just because you're writing it down. You want an accurate picture of your diet as it is now, so approximate amounts as closely as possible.

If you want to make your own, take a sheet of paper and divide it into four columns. Label the columns Meal (i.e. Breakfast, Lunch, Snack, Dinner), Food Item (include product name brand, restaurants, etc.), Quantity (g, ml, T, tsp, cup, oz, etc.), Notes: (include breakdown of food items, or ingredients of homemade meals). At the bottom of the sheet (or on another sheet of paper), mark off a place to record water intake, and record one hash mark for every 8 ounces of water.

CHAPTER 2: MOVE

Three-day activity diary

*Whatever you can do or dream you can, begin it. Boldness has genius,
power, and magic in it.*
- Goethe

BEFORE YOU CAN MAKE a suitable workout plan that you will stick to and get new results from, you need to evaluate what you are currently doing. How much exercise do you get on average? How much do you move outside of your workouts? Do you stick to your planned workouts, or is it easy to abandon them? Do you sit for long stretches of time while working? You'll find an example of the types of observations that will be helpful in making improved exercise and activity habits in your download package. In the Evaluate tracking pages, record your movement for three days. Include details, like how far from the store you parked, how many hours pass between stretch breaks at work, and how many times you take the stairs instead of the elevator in addition to time spent in formal exercise activities, what activity you engaged in, and how hard you worked. If you don't make it to the gym, include that too, and record why.

If you want to make your own MOVE tracking page, take a sheet of paper and mark off 9 sections (like a full-page tic-tac-toe board). In each section, record the following: Activity, Duration, Intensity, and Details.

MOVE: Day 1

Activity	Jog 1.5 miles
Duration	45 mins
Intensity	5-6 on scale of 4-10
Details	Treadmill, after work at gym
Activity	Stretches, forward bend, side bends
Duration	2 mins total (1 min each)
Intensity	Minimal
Details	Before am and pm coffee breaks
Activity	10,000 steps total walking today
Duration	Throughout the day
Intensity	Mixed, includes jog this evening
Details	Tracker data

This is an example of a completed MOVE diary:

CHAPTER 3: SLEEP

Three-night sleep diary

*"Sleep's what we need. It produces an emptiness in us into which
sooner or later energies flow."*
- M. John Cage

D O YOU PRIORITIZE SLEEP? How long do you spend in bed each night? Do you wake in the morning refreshed and ready to conquer the day, or do you feel as if you were dragged about by a truck while you slept, leaving you exhausted?

When recording your sleep data, include the time you lay down, the approximate time you fall asleep, and the time you wake up every day. Should you notice problems sleeping and are able to correlate them to behaviors or activities during the day, record that observation as well.

You'll be given the space to record three nights' worth of observations on the Evaluate pages with your download package. If you use a fitness tracker that records sleep data, include that as well. You will use this information to help you create a Sleep Booster plan.

If you want to make your own SLEEP tracking page, take a sheet of paper and record the following for each night: Time to Bed, Time to Wake, Total Hours, Energy Level (1 through 10), Tracker Data, and Other Observations.

<table>
<tr><td colspan="2" style="background:#404040;color:white;font-size:large">SLEEP: Day 1</td></tr>
<tr><td>Time to bed</td><td>11:30 pm</td></tr>
<tr><td>Time to sleep</td><td>12:20 am</td></tr>
<tr><td>Time to wake</td><td>6:30 am</td></tr>
<tr><td>Total hours</td><td>6 hrs 10 min</td></tr>
<tr><td>Energy level</td><td>1 2 3 4 5 6 7 8 9 10   (Circle one)</td></tr>
<tr><td>Tracker data</td><td>61% deep sleep, with one waking incident at 3:45 am</td></tr>
<tr><td>Other observations</td><td>Hard to wake up and get moving. Better after breakfast and coffee, but drowsy again around 9 am</td></tr>
</table>

This is an example of a completed SLEEP diary:

PART 4: CREATE

Develop Your Plan

CHAPTER 1: EAT

The Three Step Method

You deserve the fruits of a life lived with intention.
- Corey Jackson

YOU DON'T HAVE TO count calories on the regular, but you do need to have an idea of what your basic energy needs are for your goals. **Enter The Calculations**.

1. The Calculations

There are a variety of scientifically-verified formulas by which nutrition and fitness professionals calculate their clients' caloric needs, many of which are more complicated than this one.

Just know that, if you are of average activity, all formulas, calculations, and even caloric content of foods are guidelines with a bit of wiggle room. You won't precisely hit any caloric target, and you don't need to; you just need a deficit. With that in mind, all you really need to know are three key figures:

Resting Metabolic Rate (RMR) = your current weight x 11
Maintenance Calories (MC) = RMR + 400
Calorie target for weight loss (TWL) = MC – 600

For example, if you currently weigh 150 lbs, and want to lose weight while doing a moderate-intensity workout, your TWL would look like this:

$$RMR = 150 \text{ x } 11 = 1650$$
$$MC = 1650 + 400 = 2050$$
$$TWL = 2050—600 = 1450$$

You would need to consume a TWL of around 1450 calories per day to lose weight.

Once you have determined your TWL, you will construct a daily meal plan comprised of foods from The List in portions appropriate for your energy needs. The List organizes foods into five categories:

V1 = Primary Vegetables. Primary vegetables are your primary source of carbohydrate. They contain more fiber than starch, and are rich in nutrients yet sparse in calories. Therefore, you can eat many of them in unlimited amounts.

V2 = Secondary Vegetables and Grains. Secondary vegetables are more starch than fiber, which is why they are listed with grains. The other difference between the two is secondary vegetables are more calorically dense, which is why you'll notice that a smaller portion provides more calories than a large portion of primary vegetables.

You will notice some foods missing from this list. Highly-processed grain products such as white pastas, breads, polished (aka, white) and instant rice, instant oatmeal, and baked goods are not considered V2 foods for your daily consumption. You also won't find corn or soy products anywhere on the list. Because these products are, more often than not, detrimental to a weight-loss and fitness nutrition plan, and are considered among the most common food sensitivities. Create a lifestyle that doesn't include them regularly and you will be better served by your diet, instead of feeling trapped by it.

LP = Lean Proteins. Included in this category are lean animal proteins – meat, dairy products, and eggs. Always choose lean cuts of meat and lower-fat varieties of dairy products. Organic animal products are best. If you can only afford one organic expense, make it your dairy and eggs. While traditionally prepared soy beans can be a beneficial protein food, some studies have suggested that processed soy and soy-containing products can cause hormonal dysregulation and function as obesogens.[5]

FF = Fresh Fruits. Consume fresh and frozen varieties of fruits found in this category. Canned fruit is tricky, because it's packed with either fruit juice or syrup (read, added sugar and calories), so it should be avoided. As a rule, fruit juice is best avoided as well; it contains all of the sugar and none of the fiber of fresh fruit, which is crucial to slowing sugar absorption.

On the other end of the fruit spectrum is dried fruit, from which all the water has been removed. Thus, while dried fruit retains the fruit's fiber, it's a concentrated nugget of sugar. So it's less filling than its fresh counterpart.

HF = Healthy Fats. Healthy fats are primarily plant-based foods that are rich in naturally occurring fats. These include nuts and seeds and their butters, avocado, olives, and oils made from them. Also included in this category is fatty fish and purified fish oil supplements. This category does NOT include synthetic fats, such as trans fats; these should be avoided at all costs as they have been shown to cause cardiovascular problems.

Another helpful feature of The List is that it defines a serving, and how many calories a serving provides. Without that information, it would be easy to blissfully and ignorantly overconsume even the whole-est and healthiest of whole healthy foods.

Too much of a good thing is still too much. It's important to be aware of how much you're eating. It's easier to overeat without realizing it than it is to under-eat. For that reason, the Healthy Habits System™ Planner provides a framework for planning your meals and room to record what you eat at each meal.

HEALTHY HABITS STRATEGY:
Treat once a week

Of course, you want to create healthy meals that fit your daily meal plan AND are delicious and appealing so that you don't feel constantly pulled back to your old favorite foods. But you CAN create a healthy diet that includes the chance to indulge in a weekly treat.

Granted, if you have a sensitivity or allergy, don't indulge it; food sensitivities don't take a holiday. But treating keeps you focused and free from feeling deprived, both important strategies for maintaining motivation and forming a healthy-eating lifestyle. Keep a running list of temptations or cravings that come up during the week.

When you get to Saturday, review your list and decide which one still sounds irresistible. Then enjoy! Make it an event, and return to your satisfying, healthy meal plan without missing a beat.

Now you know how much of what foods you should be eating to achieve your health and fitness goals. (Once you've reached your goal, do the Calculations again at that weight, without the calorie deficit, for your maintenance calorie target (MCT).)

You've reviewed The List and have hopefully found many of your favorite foods, and are excited about trying new ones. If you enjoy cooking, or just love food (hands up if that's you!) the next part is fun: fitting delicious, satisfying foods into a daily meal plan that can provide room for culinary adventure and improved wellness, side by side.

Believe it! Good nutrition for weight loss and fitness maintenance can be ecstatically delicious! Even better, with proper planning and advanced preparation as a habit, good nutrition won't take over your already full life. Use the space on the next few pages to create your meal plan.

Decide what meal schedule works best for you – three meals with three snacks, or two snacks, or even one snack – and divide your servings up accordingly. Your meal schedule will depend on your energy needs as well as your regular schedule's requirements.

If you work demanding shifts that don't allow for regular breaks, you would be better served with three larger meals; if your schedule allows, you may be able to better manage hunger by incorporating two small snacks between your meals. If you work out first thing in the morning before breakfast, you should plan to consume a low-glycemic bedtime snack that is slowly absorbed to balance your glucose levels while you sleep, to facilitate repair mechanisms that occur during sleep, and to fuel your workout in the morning.

2. THE LIST

Included in your download package is the list of healthy foods used in The Healthy Habits System to help you build your meals.

3. THE LEVELS

Your task, now that you know your calorie target and what foods to eat, is to determine in which of the above Levels your calorie target lands. The Levels will guide your meal plan.

The Levels, listed on the next few pages, help you determine how many servings of each food to eat to satisfy a balanced meal plan that distributes calories from fat (25%), protein (35%), and carbohydrate (40%).

Use the Create Worksheet in your download package to (a) calculate your TWL, and (b) record your Level and how many servings of each food category you should eat.

For reference, here are the levels, along with how many servings of each food category you should target:

Level A (TWL = 1200-1399):
- V1: <= 4 Servings
- V2: 2 Servings
- LP: 4 Servings
- FF: 2 Servings
- HF: 3 Servings

Level B (TWL = 1400-1599):
- V1: <=5 Servings
- V2: 2 Servings
- LP: 5 Servings
- FF: 2 Servings
- HF: 4 Servings

Level C (TWL = 1600-1799):

- V1: <=6 servings
- V2: 2 Servings
- LP: 6 Servings
- FF: 3 Servings
- HF: 4 Servings

Level D (TWL = 1800+)

- V1: <=6 Servings
- V2: 3 Servings
- LP: 7 Servings
- FF: 3 Servings
- HF: 4 Servings

Easy peasy, lemon squeezy. Speaking of lemons – you can eat/squeeze as many lemons and limes as you want. Score! There may not be a free lunch, but there are (a short brief list of) Free Foods, and lemons and limes are found on it.

Here's the rest of the Free Foods list: (Note: In order to be considered a Free Food, the vegetables are either raw or prepared with a small amount of broth or vinegar – no cooking fats.)

- black coffee* (sweetened with stevia or xylitol)*
- bok choy
- broccoli
- celery
- collard greens
- cucumber
- kale
- lettuce
- mushrooms
- flavor extracts (ie, vanilla, almond, peppermint)
- garlic
- fresh and dried herbs
- hot sauce
- mustard
- onions
- radishes
- spinach
- sprouts
- unsalted spices
- unsweetened tea, hot or iced*
- all vinegars
- xanthan gum and arrowroot powder*

*While unsweetened coffee and black tea contribute very little to your daily caloric load, they contain caffeine, which serves as both a mild metabolic enhancer and a powerful diuretic. The former we like, unless it overstimulates or agitates you. The latter, however, must be combatted with adequate hydration; we will discuss that in the next section.

*Most artificial sweeteners should be avoided; some studies have indicated they can inflict damage on your hormone balance and metabolic rate. However, stevia, birch xylitol, and erythritol can be used in moderation with minimal impacts.

*Xanthan gum and arrowroot powder are thickening agents that can be used in lieu of cornstarch. Because corn is considered one of the most common food allergens, it or its products are not recommended for regular use in The Healthy Habits System™.

Your meal plan

How many times will you eat daily? What will you eat each time?

Whatever meal schedule you decide works for you, there is room for it in the Healthy Habits System™. Now for some specifics.

1) It's generally best practice to at least pair a carbohydrate (V1 or V2) with a protein or a healthy fat in meals and snacks.

2) Avail yourself to the abundance of V1 servings provided to all Levels, and choose unlimited veggies (those marked with a * in The List) to bulk up your meals and snacks.

3) You may also find that your blood sugar and energy levels are more balanced by consuming V2 foods in the morning or following workouts.

4) Evenly distribute protein and healthy fats through the day.

If you are not accustomed to eating at regular intervals – perhaps you get so consumed with the passion of your projects that you forget to eat until your stomach growls loud enough to penetrate your thoughts – eating on a schedule will take some getting used to. But don't worry; it won't take long before you notice the undeniable benefits of sustained mental and physical energy that you'll reap from feeding and watering yourself consistently throughout the day.

You'll also find some helpful tips and tricks in the following pages to make it easier to adopt as a routine. The sample meal schedule below, ideal for Level A, is meant for illustrative (not prescriptive) purposes. Take some time to sketch out a meal schedule for yourself in the worksheet. It can be as simple or as precise as you want.

Level A sample meal plan:
Breakfast: 1 V1, 1 V2, 1 LP
AM Snack: 1 FF, 1 LP
Lunch: 1–2 V1, 1 V2, 1 LP, 1 HF
PM Snack: 1 FF or V1
Dinner: 1–2 V1, 1 LP, 1 HF

The purpose is to help you adjust your thinking around your eating – to make it intentional instead of an afterthought pulled from a vending machine. By no means is this exercise intended to overwhelm you.

Once you have determined what meal schedule works best for your lifestyle and needs, get creative with some meal ideas for breakfast, lunch, dinner, and snacks using your favorites from The List. Use the chart in your downloaded worksheet package to jot down some ideas.

Take recipes or ideas from healthy food blogs and cookbooks, clean up family comfort-food favorites, or go crazy and innovate something entirely new! You can pull from these ideas for your weekly meal plans.

Use the Plan Worksheets to create your meal plan, and some meal ideas that incorporate your favorites from The List.

CHAPTER 2: DRINK

Your hydration strategy

Water is the driving force in nature.
- Vincent van Gogh

H OW MUCH WATER do you need? The amount varies from person to person, depending on many factors including your environment, activity level, and caffeine consumption. And it may surprise you.

First, refer to your three-day intake data for your daily water consumption. Then average those amounts together in the boxed marked Daily Hydration Average to get a general idea of how much water you're drinking now.

Daily Hydration Average
[Day 1 (............... oz) +
Day 2 (............... oz) +
Day 3 (............. oz)] ÷ 3 = ... =
your daily water average

Next, work the Hydration Equation to see how much water you should be drinking. Use an estimate, based on your intake evaluation, for how much caffeinated and/or caloric beverages (including alcohol) you consume. Remember that the figure you get here is your general hydration target. You should base your daily water intake on your exact needs each day. The daily spreads will make it easy to do that.

Hydration Equation
(your current bodyweight (#)) ÷2 +
(# caffeinated and/or caloric beverages) * 8 =
oz water goal

Many people that think they stay adequately hydrated are surprised to find, when they do this exercise, how little water they are actually drinking; this may be the case for you. Don't worry; you're not alone! And you're in for a treat; once you do make adequate hydration a habit, your body will begin operating with such efficiency that low energy, cravings, and caffeine urges will be threatened with extinction.

Hydration strategy:
Bottled water or tap?

That's totally up to you. Just make sure you are drinking plenty of clean water. If you opt for bottled water, research bottling sources to make sure you are purchasing clean water. If you opt for tap, make sure you are filtering it to remove unwanted contaminants.

CHAPTER 3: MOVE

Using your worksheets to create your Fitness Strategy

Remove the limits from your mind and open up a path of endless possibilities in your fitness.
- Corey Jackson

USING THE INFORMATION you gathered in Create, let's get started building your Move plan. This is definitely a part of the plant that most impacts your day-to-day schedule, so really give it some thought as you go through this section, and consider how this is going to fit into your routine, and what may have to give.

1. First, list activities you enjoy or want to try in each of the four facets of your Healthy Habits System™ Optimal Fitness Strategy.

2. Next, consider the List of Dreams and Goals you made in DO. What are the big, scary some-day things that you've always wanted to experience, but have never felt like you were fit enough for? Do you want to hike in and out of the Grand Canyon? Run the Boston Marathon? Enter an amateur physique competition?

You hold within you the power to accomplish anything you passionately desire. Barring any physical limitation, the frameworks provided in this workbook can help you achieve any goal you set for yourself.

So now's the time to start making plans; some-day is finally within reach! List below any Dream List items you're ready to start checking off. Compare them to the activities you listed to the left. Can any of those prepare you to achieve them?

3. Now, craft these aspects into a weekly plan that is fun, fits your life, and takes you toward your big, scary Dream List experience by putting them together into a daily and weekly schedule. Remember that specificity is imperative when it comes to creating frameworks for success.

Schedule your training when nothing else will interfere. Adjust your schedule to accommodate your workouts by eliminating activities that can be, and by shifting things that can't. Obviously some things are non-negotiable. Likely your work schedule is one of those. If you are a student, your class schedule is definitely predefined for you. Family obligations may be beyond your control. And you must carve out and protect 7–9 hours each 24-hour cycle for sleep. So look to things you can negotiate: television time, for instance. Cut corners in certain routines to shave off time. Share responsibilities with team members and family members.

The point is, as we discussed in DO, the things that are important to you have a way of making room for themselves. Facilitate prioritizing your workouts by making them a permanent part of your week.

CHAPTER 4: SLEEP

Your sleep booster strategy.

To achieve the impossible dream, try going to sleep.
- Joan Klempner

RECORD YOUR Sleep Booster Plan on the corresponding worksheet. Everyone should start by turning down their lights 2–3 hours before going to bed, which optically triggers the production and release of melatonin, the neurotransmitter that induces sleep. Almost equally important is the screen curfew, as most digital screens emit a spectrum of blue light that disrupts melatonin secretion. So while we may doze off while watching television, our sleep quality is insufficient as it lacks adequate melatonin support.

Work back eight hours from when you need to rise each morning to determine your bedtime. Then, work back one hour to establish a sufficient screen curfew, and three hours to when you should begin dimming the lights and calming your brain before sleep. Add as many Sleep Booster Behaviors as possible, particularly those involving a bedtime routine and ideal sleep environment. Each day throughout the planner you'll be tracking what you Eat (and whether it was planned), Drink, how you Move, and your Sleep observations, along with which Sleep Boosters you applied.

Often when establishing healthy habits in order to transform your health and your body, you must simply trust the process long enough to begin seeing results (see Troubleshooting on page 45 to know when blind faith isn't enough). Sleep is different, though. You might need to experiment with Sleep Booster combinations until you find one that consistently works well for you, and that experimentation should begin right away.

Approach your sleep as a scientist conducting an important investigation. Your mission is to create the most scientifically-sound sleep boosting program possible using good experimental technique, which requires proper data collection as well as objective analysis and Sleep Booster testing.

If you find that a select few Sleep Boosters work to encourage optimal sleep, that is all you need. You may find you need to implement several or all of the Sleep Booster Behaviors. If, however, your established bedtime routine combined with the right sleep environment does not result in consistent optimal sleep, ensure you are avoiding the Sleep Disruptor Behaviors. If all is in place there, begin by adding one of the Sleep Booster Supplements until you establish the proper regimen for your optimal sleep efficiency.

Making a SMART Goal and Action Plan.

A goal without a plan is just a wish.

Setting goals and creating healthy habits go together. Having a goal, a purpose to work toward, is great incentive to build habits and rituals. These things make you more likely to achieve what you've set out to do. Before you set out on a journey, you need to know where you are going. How will you know how far you've traveled if you don't mark the start and end?

There are some tools in your download package that will help you with this. The first is the SMART Goal System. A SMART goal is one that is Specific, Measurable, Achievable, Relevant and Time-bound. We could spend several pages discussing this topic, but it's easy once you see it. Here are two examples of goals, one SMART, and the other not:

Not SMART: Be a better swimmer. (This is a nice thing to want, but the goal isn't SMART.)

SMART: Improve 100m backstroke time by 5 seconds by the end of 4 weeks through attention to stroke consistency, breathing and body position.

Can you see how the second goal is better? It would be impossible to fail the first goal because there isn't an objective measure. According to the SMART model, a goal you can't fail is a goal you can't succeed at either.

Let's do one together:
SMART Goal: Lose 10 lbs. by the end of 28 days, by focusing on consistent exercise, and eating on-plan each day, using an intended 400 calorie/day deficit for the four weeks.

Key actions/habits: To accomplish this, I will need to be in the gym every morning except Sundays, every week, and will need to consistently grocery shop, precook and package planned meals so that I can eat only what I have determined to eat for 28 days. Time commitment: I will work out one hour per day (six hours/week). This will need to be at 5:30 am, as I must be ready and on the road by 7:00 to make it to work on time. Bedtime will need to be earlier than normal. I will need to set aside 3 to 4 hours on the weekends for meal planning, shopping and pre-cooking. (I cook anyway, so this should help alleviate some time elsewhere in the week.)

Self: I will need to start winding down earlier at night, and will have to give up my 9 pm glass of wine and 10 pm TV show for the 28 days.

People: I will need to enlist the help of my family, particularly my spouse who is used to watching TV and drinking a glass of wine with me in the evenings. This will need to be a team effort. I don't expect my boss to be okay with me being late, so I will need to go to bed at 9:30 each night so I can get up at 5:00 every morning.

Surroundings: I have some space on my cube wall I can hang up my meal plan, and will probably get some motivational quotes or photos to keep there to help me stay the course on tough days when I want to raid the snack machine.

Financial Cost: I'm expecting my grocery bill to go up a little, especially the first week. However, we've agreed to not buy wine for the four weeks, and decided to cancel one of our streaming TV subscriptions for the month to offset the cost. (We won't be watching the shows anyway.)

Milestones: Every day, I will put a star on my meal plan at work if I end the day having eaten on-plan. I will set workout goals each week to keep me motivated to Move. I will weigh and measure at the beginning of the program, and at the end of each week to see if I'm making progress. If I'm going to do this, I need to lose 2.5lbs per week, so I'll need to see how I'm doing along the way. I won't make big changes unless I get to the end of two weeks and haven't lost any weight.

The next tool is the Fishbone Diagram, and it's a way of visualizing cause and effect. It can be used either to diagnose a problem, or to identify the necessary inputs and influences to generate a desired outcome. To use this tool, look at the words in the pre-populated circles, and brainstorm as many words as you can that you believe directly contribute to success in that area. If you find something that tends to detract from success there, draw a circle around it so you can see it as something you need to watch out for. Connect the lines with arrows (denoting contributing factors to your success), like the example found in your download package.

CHAPTER 5: TROUBLESHOOTING YOUR PLAN

*But one thing is for sure: No matter how organized we are, or how
well we plan, we can always expect the unexpected.*
- Brandon Jenner

LET'S SET THE RECORD straight: *Weight loss in any form does not follow a linear progression.* You are probably aware of that, if only on a subconscious level, especially if you have attempted weight loss before. It is impossible to correctly predict or control the timeline of your fat loss on your plan.

What you can control is your attitude about the process and your efforts and behaviors throughout. It is exponentially more beneficial to focus on your behaviors – doing the stuff – than to focus on your results – the way your body responds to the stuff. And while you need to measure your progress by taking weight and body measurements weekly, resist the temptation to tamper with the plan or give up before you have reached your goals if your fat loss is not progressing according to your preconceived ideas.

Often, what it comes down to is a matter of trust. You have to trust the process, your plan, and yourself. The best way to do that is to make sure you are actually following your plan. Above all else, The Healthy Habits System™ was written to help you pay attention to your habits, to enable you to live with intention. It provides a framework that will help you lose weight, if you are properly following the plan you make with it.

While you are establishing your habits, you will have to focus your intention on it. Once these behaviors are ingrained in your life so that they are automatic, you won't have to micromanage – *they will be habits* - but until then, exercise tight control over your behaviors. The tighter your control, the more you can trust yourself and your plan – and you will achieve results. Following are areas of control to check when your plan is getting a lackluster response.

EAT

If you feel you aren't shedding fat at a reasonable pace – about 2 pounds per week on average – make sure you are actually eating according to your plan.

First, ensure you are minding your portions, particularly of healthy fats (HF) and starch and grain (V2) foods. Weigh and measure your food to make sure you're not fudging your serving sizes up. Next, make sure you're eating ample fresh vegetables (V1). Beyond vitamins and minerals, the phytonutrients and enzymes provided by V1 foods fuel your metabolism so much so that skipping them is detrimental to your progress. You can control fats by opting for raw or steamed vegetables, or sautéing with a combination of broths and vinegars.

Don't skip fruit (FF), but do skip the higher-glycemic options. Choose instead berries (blueberries, strawberries, blackberries, raspberries, etc.), grapefruits, tart green apples, and pears over grapes, bananas, and tropical fruits. Weigh lean protein (LP) portions, and choose lean cuts of unprocessed meats. It may be beneficial to eliminate dairy choices for a while; just make sure you take a calcium supplement when you do.

Finally, choose the least-processed foods on The List. Whole-grain crackers, breads, and cereals are on The List, but if consuming these foods keeps you from seeing the results you want, replace them with unprocessed whole food options such as quinoa and sweet potatoes.

Pay attention along the way to how your body responds to the food you eat. It is possible that some amount of your struggle is due to water retention. Processed starches can contribute to that. Nutrient timing can also impact water retention and fat burning; consume your starches in your post-workout meal or snack to minimize these problems.

If you struggle with bloating and digestive issues such as constipation, curb your salt intake and make sure you are adequately hydrating. Which brings us to...

DRINK

Use the Hydration Equation to establish your water baseline. If you limit salt while drinking your water baseline and you're still retaining water, increase your water consumption by 8–12 ounces per day until you visit the bathroom at least one time per hour. Stay amply hydrated throughout your workouts, including Active Rest activities. If you are still experiencing water retention, it may be time to see your doctor.

MOVE

Be honest with yourself: How intensely are you exercising? Rate your efforts on a scale of 1–10. If you can still talk during your Sweat sessions, you are exercising between a 5 and 6; if you can only utter short phrases without stopping to catch your breath, you're at 7 or 8; if you are going at a pace that you can only sustain for a minute or less, you are exercising at a 10. If you could do more than 10–15 repetitions of any strength exercise with little muscle burn and fatigue, you are exercising at a 6 or lower; if you can complete no more than 10 reps with good form, you have completed a level-10 set.

Obviously, you can't maintain a solid 10 for the duration of a workout, but you should aim to hit a 10 at least a couple of times (and the more the better) during each session. Intensity is important in Sweat and Strength workouts, and can be increased by increasing your speed and resistance, decreasing rest between high-intensity work, or a combination of these.

If you are finding it difficult to achieve Level 10 intensity with a certain mode of exercise, switch things up. For example, if running is too hard on your knees to achieve a 10, try cycling or rowing. If you've been using resistance bands and haven't hit a 10 by your 20th rep, switch to weight training. The more intense your workouts, the more your body will respond to them. And one of those enhanced responses will likely be in your sleep efficiency.

SLEEP

Are you going to bed an hour or more before midnight? Are you sleeping through the night? Or are you sacrificing sleep to make time for work or workouts?

Efficient sleep is crucial for proper recovery from workouts as well as adequate hormone release for optimal fat loss, so your sleep quality cannot be ignored. Continue adjusting your schedule and your Sleep Booster routine until you can report high energy levels for several consecutive mornings.

It can be tempting to panic and switch plans midstream when you feel you aren't getting results. But resist that urge by considering that, just maybe, it's been a contributor to yo-yo weight loss/gain patterns in your past. The only way to form solid, lifetime healthy habits is to perform them consistently. Consistency is also the key to weight loss success. Funny how that word keeps coming up.

CHIEF PLANNER TIP:

Make sure you're flexing

Flexibility is a crucial part of Move; it's important to your results, so be sure you take the time to work on it. Warm up properly before Sweat and Strength, and stretch before and after. Incorporate at least one yoga session or other form of long Flex training. Doing so will decrease your recovery time between high-intensity workouts, protect your muscles and joints from injury, and allow you to burn calories – and fat – when you Move at a higher rate.

DO YOUR PLAN

Knowledge is of no value unless you put it into practice
- Anton Chekhov

AT THIS POINT, you've learned the System. Now is the time to put it into action! There are enough planning sheets in your download package (remember your code from the Introduction) to allow you to get started and to learn the system.

Take your before photos and adhere them to the Tracking page. Come back to the workbook when you need help or forget something. This is a LOT to learn in a short time, so don't feel bad if you feel lost. Just refer to the relevant sections, or even go online and ask for help at info@prettygoodplanners.com.

After the Four Weeks are done, take your AFTER photos, and prepare to be amazed at the progress you see! Then come back and continue in the next chapter: RE-EVALUATE.

You got this!!

EPILOGUE: WHAT NEXT?

Practical Advice for Sustained Results

RE-EVALUATE

Where Actions Become Habits

*Our goals can only be reached through a vehicle of a plan, in which
we must fervently believe, and upon which we must vigorously act.
There is no other route to success.*
 - Pablo Picasso

FOUR WEKS. For twenty-eight days, you have lived your new healthy habits. You kicked your bad habits to the curb and replaced them with a system that ensures your success.

Twenty. Eight. Days.

Good on you! Seriously, high fives all around. You may be wondering, what now? After all, that's the question most people ask when they get to the end of a diet or a program. As a former member of the 80%, you have likely asked the same question yourself. If you have previous experience with weight loss reversion, you likely see maintenance as an elusive dream state – that you've never fully attained. But this time is different.

Tomorrow should look pretty much like today, and the day before that. The day after tomorrow? Yep, the same. You didn't just work a plan, you created a new set of habits that you can use to take you into a permanently healthy lifestyle. You ensured that you included foods you enjoy and you were not deprived of your favorites. You chose to do only activities that get you jazzed up because you love them so and can't imagine life without them. You've discovered the wondrous benefits of drinking enough water, and regular restorative sleep.

So now, continue living your healthy habits. Make sure you have your Healthy Habits System™ 90-Day Planner, and keep going!

Keep planning and precooking your meals, allowing that habit to diminish the stress of dinner on busy nights. Keep drinking your water, practicing joyful movement and resting blissfully.

But first, take a moment to evaluate your current position on your journey toward fulfilling the goals you set out to achieve four weeks ago. Use the Re-Evaluate worksheet to help you in this process. Reference your SMART goal and Fishbone exercises while working through it.

• Have you achieved all you wanted to? Good for you! Recalculate your calorie needs without a deficit, and set your servings level accordingly. Keep planning your meals. Aim higher in your workouts and keep crushing them. The habits you've made through this four weeks will help you maintain your progress and live at your goals. And if you have yet to start checking items off of your Dream List (see Create: Move), now's the time to go for it!

• Do you have further to go? Great! You've taken the time needed to lay a proper foundation for your progress. *Success is predetermined by your ability to maintain these habits.* Recalculate your calorie needs and adjust your servings level accordingly. If you are still progressing – steady as she goes! However, if your progress has slowed and/or plateaued, this may be the perfect opportunity to tighten things up to break through. Not all calories come from foods that treat your body the same, so make sure you're getting your calories from nutrient-rich whole foods.

• Revisit Troubleshooting your Plan and determine how you can tighten up your hold on the reigns.

1. Evaluate your meals to make sure you are making the best choices. If higher glycemic starches and fruits make up any of your FF and V2 servings, switch them out for low-glycemic options. If you haven't already, invest in a food scale to weigh your portions. Exercising more diligent control may be what you need going forward. However, before

you cut calories even more, look to other means of increasing your caloric deficit, by your activity.

2. Does your fitness plan still fit your needs, or are you finding it a little lackluster? Don't give up on it or settle for boring workouts. If you allow boredom to creep in, chances are you will also allow your intensity (and thus your fat-burning potential) to wane as well. *Always be committed to finding your workout Muse.*

3. Outside of the gym, there are areas in which you can move more and burn more, and that might be just what you need if you are experiencing a plateau. Use an activity tracker to make sure you're walking enough. Set it so that it triggers you to get up and stretch every hour while you're working. Always take the stairs instead of the elevator, park far away from the entrance, and choose to walk the extra blocks when you have time instead of waiting for the bus or calling an Uber. *This added activity can contribute even more to your caloric deficit than your diet.* Fitness professionals refer to the caloric expenditure from every-day activity as Non-Exercise Activity Thermogenesis (NEAT for short).

4. Did you set a performance goal? That big, crazy, Dream-List caliber physical adventure you want to have? How's training going for that? Re-assess your plan and see if you're still on track to achieve your dreams. If you haven't yet, it's time to schedule at least the first step towards that goal. A marathon? Sign up for a 10K, or a half-marathon. A mountain-climbing expedition? Schedule a climbing trip and start planning. Life is meant to be lived! Make sure you do the thing that excites you. Make sure you never look back on your life with regret for the things you never did! Whatever it is, keep working your Healthy Habit System™ toward making it happen.

RECALIBRATE.

*Visions don't change, they are only refined. … Be stubborn about the
vision, but flexible with your plan.*
- John C. Maxwell

O nce you've entered maintenance, it is still important to remain vigilant against weight regain. Even healthy habits, once they become routine, are subject to drift. With your focus on other things – work, school, family – it is not uncommon for your portions to begin expanding ever so slightly, or for you to become relaxed in your hydrating diligence. It can become too easy to just go through the motions of your daily workouts, or begin cutting into them to allow time for other things. The best way to guard against the subconscious sabotage that can happen during maintenance is to reassess regularly. Likely the most powerful tip anyone could give you now is this: Commit to living with intention. Don't just let life happen to you; no, you make life happen on your terms!

The best habit you can develop is Living on Purpose. Check in with yourself regularly. Keep your finger on the pulse. Pay diligent attention to how your clothes fit. Set a boundary weight for yourself; weigh yourself regularly, and take measures to ensure that your weight doesn't crawl up beyond it.

Assess your moods and your energy levels regularly; if you begin to feel listless and exhausted, take inventory of your sleep efficiency and evaluate your Sleep Booster habits. By living with intention, you will be able to live in the confidence that rightfully belongs to those that are in charge – because you will be. And if you find that your pants have gotten a bit snugger, commit to a period of focused recalibration. View it as a practice, like yoga or meditation. Sometimes it takes the reset of intense focus to realize how far we've slipped from optimal health. If you are dedicated to using your 90-day planner and recalibrating your habits and goals once a quarter, you'll catch any possible slide before it becomes a full-on rebound. These two practices will help you remain among the successful

20% of maintainers. Again, congratulations for committing to your health by changing your habits! Welcome to your new, liberated life, structured on a Healthy Habits™ framework.

[1] Ng, Marie et al. Global, regional, and national prevalence of overweight and obesity in children and adults during 1980–2013: a systematic analysis for the Global Burden of Disease Study 2013. *The Lancet*, August 2014. Volume 384, No. 9945, p766–781, 30.

[2] Wing, RR., Phelan, S. Long-term weight loss maintenance. *American Journal of Clinical Nutrition*, 2005 Jul;82(1 Suppl):222S-225S.

[3] Lally,P., van Jaarsveld, C., Potts, H., Wardle, J. How are habits formed: Modelling habit formation in the real world. *European Journal of Social Psychology*. October 2010, Volume 40, Issue 6, pages 998–1009.

[iv] Look for less-refined fish oil supplements, with a good balance of EPA and DHA. Barleans produces an excellent liquid product which can be found at health food and supplement stores, or online at http://www.barleans.com/.

[v] The National Healthy Sleep Awareness Project has published this study and a lot of helpful information at http://www.sleepeducation.org/healthysleep;0.

[vi] Have your doctor run a blood panel for Vitamin D and other nutrient deficiencies before you start supplementing.

[vii] Recommended reading: Sleep Smarter by Shawn Stevenson. http://sleepsmarterbook.com/.